Aunt Carrie's Guide to a Long, Healthy and Happy Life, the Natural, Low Cost Way

I'm not a doctor, nurse, nutritionist or other health care professional. However, I learned at my mother's knee how to stay healthy and live a long life, on a budget. Grandma Helen was far from wealthy and in fact was the youngest of five children who were raised by their hard-working single mother (when the father was above all a good provider) abandoned by their poppa. You might say that Grandma Helen was dirt poor most of her life.

Not blessed with the benefit of higher education, Grandma Helen read everything she could about nutrition. When other kids were eating instant puddings, pop tarts and other sugary treats, my typical dessert would be jell-o with grated carrots. Sack lunches consisted of granola, yogurt, apples, not potato chips. Oh, how I hated being different!

And sodas? Sprite and 7-Up when we were too sick to eat – and to this day those citrusy drinks make me feel nauseated – and a small glass of Coca Cola as a special, really special, treat.

When we did have a dessert, it was homemade and chocolate, never sugar pie (sugar, flour, milk). "If I'm going to eat a sweet, I'm not going to waste it. It has to be good." Grandma Helen knew best, and Grandma Helen ruled the kitchen with a firm hand.

You might have guessed that all this food control turned me into a rebel. As soon as I was able to get out and about, I bought Pepsi, hiding it in the trunk of my car. I later switched to The Real Thing after a doctor recommended it for a tummy troubles and became addicted to the sugar-caffeine combo. I can stop any time, just ask me. I've quit many, many times, once for several years.

However, when I recently was felled by a strain of flu (I could not tell you the last time I was sick), Coca Cola was all that I could hold down, and it is a very limited aspect part of my healthy living program.

During my rebellious period I ate doughnuts, candy bars, anything sweet. The more I ate, the more I craved.

After being suddenly single, I longed to meet Mr. Right. However, no one that I liked found me attractive. I was "too fat." I'm still not svelte, but after the humiliation of being rejected I decided to ditch the processed sugar for fruit. Sugar is sugar, you might say, but the natural sugars in fruit satisfy me better than candy. I lost weight and feel better (as in younger). My skin is smoother and wrinkles seem to be avoiding me.

These tips are common sense, easily obtainable rules to live by. There aren't going to be suggestions that you buy exotic fruit, maintain a killer exercise regimen or do anything that isn't readily available to most people.

Aunt Carrie's Tip #1: Eat more fruits and vegetables and less food of limited nutritional value. Yes, we all know this, but let's burn into our brains and follow this plan of attack against growing old too soon.

Eat healthy 80% of the time and allow yourself a few indiscretions.

Although not strictly speaking a smoothie, this drink is a refreshing healthy alternative to soda. Start with orange or pineapple juice, watered down a little if you prefer, and add a ripe banana. This is the base.

Depending upon what I have on hand, I toss in any combination of a few fresh strawberries, pieces of watermelon, cantaloupe, papaya, or mango, or chilled crushed pineapple and run it through a small blender. I don't use ice cubes and never ever add yogurt, although I love it other ways. If mint is in season, a few sprigs go in. Sprinkle with a little cinnamon or ginger if you have it. My niece, also Grandma Helen's protégé in matters of health, likes kale in her health drink. Go a little crazy!

Grandma Helen kept bananas in the house and often joked that a monkey would be happy living with her. I make it a habit to eat at least one a day, usually in my faux smoothie (above).

Among other things, bananas and most other fruits, fight the onset of macular degeneration. They also help prevent strokes and reduce blood pressure and battle depression. (Bananas along with exercise and prayer/meditation are my first line to sustain my mental health)

There are many practical uses for lemons. One woman who still worked part-time well into her eighties credited her morning drink of one tablespoon of honey, one tablespoon of lemon juice in a small glass of hot water for her near perfect attendance record.

Grandma Helen put lemon slices or lemon juice in her drinks to help control her blood pressure. The scent of lemon is a mood lightener and God knows, we all can use a little of that these days.

Cinnamon aids in digestion and is thought to lower blood sugar. If you take medication to treat diabetes consult your doctor before adding it to your diet. I sprinkle cinnamon over most desserts and stir it into hot chocolate. It not only adds flavor but it also seems to calm my appetite.

Grandma Helen drank tomato juice instead of sugary soda. I still drink a can or two a day, but I have also incorporated tomato juice into my every day life. It's good chilled, and it's tasty microwaved for a minute. Add minced onions, black pepper, and fresh basil and you have a low calorie soup. I also prepare rice in a half tomato juice-half water mixture.

Grandma Helen celebrated her British roots by drinking several cups of tea, sweetened with a teaspoon of honey, every day of her long life.

Grandma Helen ate a bit of dark chocolate daily along with a banana to help control her blood pressure. I eat dark chocolate for health reasons but confess I prefer milk chocolate.

Watermelon was another of Grandma Helen's pleasures and it also helped regulate blood pressure.

Berries and citrus fruits are other healthy yet tasty treats. Low in calories and high in Vitamin C, they are a mainstay of my nutritional plan.

Garlic is said to boost immunity, fight off aging, and promote heart health. Mince it fine enough and even finicky eaters won't notice. Garlic is one of my go-tos. Cinnamon gets tossed into anything sweet, and anything else gets doctored up with garlic and red pepper flakes. I also add cilantro when I have it in the house.

Pomegranates are a relatively new addition to my refrigerator and I admit it took me awhile to figure out how to eat them. I also drink pomegranate juice when it is on sale (it seems expensive otherwise). Pomegranates help prevent hardening of the arteries.

Musk melons (cantaloupes) reduce "bad" cholesterol.

They are also an inexpensive delicacy. I like to eat half a melon right out of the fridge, and sometimes add a little whipped topping.

Grandma Helen drank a small cup of cranberry juice cocktail every morning. She also made cranberry sauce for Thanksgiving and Christmas dinners. She would have none of the canned stuff – it had to be homemade. If you are not included to make your own, some grocery deli departments have old fashioned homemade cranberry sauce.

Yogurt is a probiotic ("for life") that may help reduce the risk of high blood pressure and osteoporosis. It contains protein, calcium, potassium, magnesium, and Vitamin B-2 and B-12.

Although yogurt is sometimes used to sooth irritated vaginal tissues, I do not know if Grandma Helen used it for that purpose. Talking about it would have been just plain weird.

Raisin Bran Banana Muffins

Grandma Helen ate these regularly, and for once, I baked them. This is my own version.   .

3 ripe bananas

1 egg

¼ cup honey

1/2 cup milk

3 Tablespoons butter or vegetable oil

1 1/2 cup raisin bran cereal

1 cup flour

1 apple, cored and minced

2 teaspoons baking powder

1/4 tsp. baking soda

1/4 tsp. Nutmeg, cinnamon or pumpkin pie spice

Preheat oven to 400 degrees. Grease muffin tin. In medium bowl combine all ingredients except raisin bran, flour, baking powder and baking soda; let sit for a few minutes. Combine dry ingredients and stir in until moist. Bake 25 minutes.

You can substitute up to ½ cup whole wheat flour for white as long as flour totals 1 cup.

I add fresh blueberries when I have them.

Fresh Tomato-Cucumber Salad

2 beefsteak tomatoes, thinly sliced

1/4 red onion, thinly sliced

1 cucumber, thinly sliced

2 Tablespoons extra-virgin olive oil, about

2 Tablespoons red wine vinegar

Mozzarella cheese, cut into thick slices or chunks

Coarse salt and black pepper

Any combination of fresh basil, oregano and cilantro leaves, dill sprigs.

Sprinkle tomatoes, cucumbers, mozzarella cheese and onions with olive oil, red wine vinegar and seasonings. Let stand about 20 minutes.

Salmon Patties

1 can salmon

Parsley flakes to taste

Salt and pepper (Grandma Helen never used salt and neither do I but some folks swear by it – I swear at it for the damage it does to my blood pressure)

2 eggs

Crushed crackers (Grandma Helen used saltines but I like the buttery kind)

1 Tablespoon minced onions

Red pepper flakes to taste (since they are alleged to speed up metabolism and alleviate pain I use them in almost everything I cook)

Drain salmon, removing bones and any skin; mash with fork; stir in eggs, minced onions, parsley, black pepper and red pepper flakes. Add enough crushed crackers to make a firm patty. Patties should not be dry. Fry in skillet with a little olive or vegetable oil; cook until golden brown; flip and fry until other side is also browned. I serve with horseradish sauce and dill sprigs.

Watermelon-Cucumber Juice

For a refreshing drink on a hot day, cut part of a watermelon and two cucumbers into chunks. Place in large pitcher, fill with water, and top with mint leaves. I thought I didn't like cucumbers until I tasted this.

Green Drink

Grandma Helen's grandson and my #1 (and only) son fixes this drink for his family and himself. It's lower calorie and lower sugar than my smoothies:

Into blender or smoothie maker:
1 cup spinach
1 cup kale
1/2 cucumber if he has it in the house
1 apple
A little chopped celery

½ teaspoon lime or lemon juice (optional)

1 teaspoon honey (optional)

Enough water to fill the container

Blend well. Sprinkle with ground ginger. This drink is an acquired taste but well worth the effort.

Grandma Helen's Cranberry Sauce

12-ounce bag fresh cranberries into a saucepan

1 cup sugar

1 strip orange zest

2 Tablespoons water

2 Tablespoons chopped celery

2 Tablespoons chopped walnuts

Pinch of salt, if desired

Pinch of cinnamon (optional)

Stir together cranberries, sugar, zest and water and

cook over low heat. Stir occasionally so that the sugar dissolves. Continue cooking until cranberries burst. Remove from heat; add celery, walnuts, salt and cinnamon; place in serving bowl and refrigerate. While growing up, it was my job to first pour bag of cranberries into a bowl filled with water and pick out any puckered berries.

Dried Beans

Dried beans lower cholesterol, reduce the risk of heart disease, stabilize blood sugar, and prevent constipation.

Grandma Helen had a go-to meal consisting of dried beans (she varied the dish by combining several types - black bean, Boston navy bean, chickpeas, great Northern bean, pinto beans and kidney beans) and chicken, two of her favorite foods.

This is her recipe for jambalaya.

In a large saucepan, bring water to boil; add a pound of dried beans; continue boiling. Boil 3 to 5 minutes; cover pan; remove from heat; let rest at room temperature for an hour; drain, rinse.

2 cups cooked beans

2 pounds skinless chicken breasts, cut into pieces

1 can diced tomatoes (no-salt)

1/4 cup chopped onion

1/4 cup chopped celery

2 to 3 gloves garlic, minced

1 cup tomato juice

Cook chicken in enough water to cover until tender. Add tomatoes, onion, celery, garlic and tomato juice and bring mixture to a boil.

Reduce heat; add beans; simmer for 10 to 15 minutes.

Serve over rice. (Grandma Helen preferred brown rice, but I like white.) Sprinkle with fresh parsley or dried parsley flakes.

Do It Yourself Yogurt (in a thermos)

1 pint whole milk

1 tablespoon live yogurt (buy a small container of plain yogurt containing live cultures)

1 Tablespoon vanilla extract

Scald milk (180 degrees F); cool to 110 degrees. Stir in 1 Tablespoon yogurt. Pour into a thermos and leave overnight (8 to

10 hours). Pour into individual containers. If desired, put jam or chocolate shavings at the bottom of container before pouring in yogurt. Refrigerate.

Grandma Helen and I made yogurt many, many times. It is very simple.

Natural painkillers include glucosamine and chondroitin which reduce arthritis pain. I take a supplement occasionally and give biscuits containing glucosamine to my elderly dog twice a day.

To soothe an earache, nuke a garlic clove for 15 seconds, remove, rub lightly with mentholated petroleum jelly and put inside your ear canal.

After hurting my foot recently (by dropping a heavy glass pitcher on my big toe) I learned that soaking in a mixture of hot water and Epsom salts not only lessens the pain but is relaxing. I soak my feet in a plastic dish tub ($1), then when the mixture cools pour over my garden. I don't use a formula; just toss a handful of salt into hot as I can stand water and soak until the water cools down.

I came down with shingles after being bullied at work and credit two things to my recovery: getting immediate treatment and the inclusion of capsaicin into my daily diet. Capsaicin readily available as it is present in hot peppers. Capsaicin also relieves arthritis pain and is credited as an appetite suppressant.

Heart Healthy Foods:

Oatmeal

Salmon

Tuna

Carrots

Blueberries

Oranges

Beans

Spinach

Broccoli

Walnuts

Brown rice

Sweet potatoes (Grandma Helen fixed them very simply: baked and topped with a little butter and sometimes brown sugar and cinnamon. She turned her nose up at the marshmallow fluff-sweet potato casserole.)

Asparagus (Grandma Helen grew asparagus for years and considered it a delicacy.)

Tomatoes (who doesn't love tomatoes?!)

Musk melon (cantaloupe)

Acorn squash (I don't remember my mother eating acorn squash but two years ago I planted a packet of seeds to see what they would do and became a huge fan of this cute little squash. Cut it in half, place it cut side down on a cookie sheet, bake for 45 minutes or until soft. Butter and a few sprinkles of brown sugar and cinnamon make this a healthy, sweet treat – almost a dessert.)

Aunt Carrie's Tip #2: Exercise. You don't have to run marathons and you should never work out to the point of exhaustion and/or emaciation. When in her nineties, every day Grandma Helen walked briskly back and forth through the hallway of her home a certain number of times, then lifted weights (two large tomato juice cans).

Get up and move around. If you are overweight, arthritic, or bedfast, do what you can do. If you can walk, walk, working up to it slowly if necessary. If you can't walk, move your arms. If you can't move your arms, then wiggle your fingers. Do whatever you can do, remembering to start out in baby steps and gradually progress.

I am sixty-five years old (and only for you would I admit that) and my main exercise is – drum roll, please – hiking. For safety's sake, I joined a hiker's group, but four to five miles is my limit, and many of the other hikers can go six, nine, up to fifteen miles in rugged terrain. I attend hikes within my range and so far have enjoyed two All Hallow's Eve walks through Green Lawn Cemetery (Ohio's second largest graveyard), a three mile walk up a steep and rocky slope with three men young enough to be my son (and I kept up), a four mile trek up a closed to the public prehistoric Indian mound with four other young men (again, I kept up) and an organized hike through a metro park off trail (where I tripped over vines three different times and became quite embarrassed when people asked if I needed help getting up).

During extreme heat, I walk in an above ground pool. Cold rain seems to seep into my bones, so I either walk around a super store or I stay home during dreary weather. Resting is important to health and longevity, too. Sometimes when I feel lazy, I remember my mother's efforts to stay active and force myself to move.

In cool, dry weather I tramp up and down elevated paved paths wandering up and down the meandering streets of our local necropolis for up to ninety minutes, as the spirit moves me. All that huffin' and puffin' gets my heart pumpin'. Why a cemetery? Even though no place is absolutely safe these days, there are often other people hiking in the area – and there are usually no dogs running loose.

A lifelong dog lover and animal rescuer, I always believed that canines smell fear and attack only those who aren't comfortable around them. Until the famous Tootsie incident that is. I was walking briskly down the side of the road when a German Shepherd came out of his yard, barking and growling – at me. I love dogs! What on earth was happening? When Tootsie lunged toward my neck, I involuntarily blocked him with my leg. Tootsie took a bite through my heavy work pants, then ran back to his yard. A member of the family called him and told me he had never bitten anyone. The family member did not offer a ride home or to call paramedics or enquire about my injury or even apologize.

I did not call the police, and I did not go to the hospital. I later learned from a neighbor that Tootsie had indeed bitten before.

Walking alone can be dangerous, as you well know, and it is smart to stay alert against threats from predators, both two and four footed as well as slithering ones.

Dress appropriately, pack mace or pepper spray (on one of the above mentioned hikes, one of the younger men assured me he was "carrying" mostly to protect us from animals but also against potential threats from humans), stay aware of your surroundings and weather conditions, and always, always, always have a fully charged cell phone in hand. Also keep in mind that cell service is zero in some forests and other areas.

Need more inspiration?

Last Mother's Day my kids surprised me with a three wheel bicycle and helmet, along with the admonition that I am to ride only on bike paths and never by myself. It is tough going, but I am now up to seven miles.

My daughter had been sedentary and sickly most of her life until she bought herself a bike and advertised for a biking buddy. She rides for ten miles whenever she has time and sleeps better, has fewer aches and pains, and is healthier and happier than ever. Grandma Helen would be so proud.

At the age of thirty my son began studying tae kwon do. His new regiment got him back into shape and also helps him deal with his stressful job and the responsibilities of having a developmentally disabled child.

Energize yourself with the exercise of your choice. Even ten or fifteen minutes will revitalize you.

If you sit at a desk for a living, get up from your work station and walk around.

My problem area – and most of us have at least one – is my abdomen, waist, midsection. Not only is it hard to find clothes to fit, but it is not healthy to carry weight there. Sit-ups seem to strengthen my back more than trim my front but it also helps me stand up straight. Side bends work for some people, but not as well as for others. My new work-out, should I accept the challenge, is something from our childhoods: a hulu hoop. I didn't master it then, but I'm going to give it my best effort now. It's cheap and it's convenient. Crank up some good ol' rock and roll and have some fun.

I confess that I don't have time (or am not able to make time) to drive to a gym and work out and for that reason am considering buying a contraption or two, and using them, not just buying them and letting them sit, to help my fitness goals. Exercise bicycles and treadmills are favorites of people who work out in home gyms.

Aunt Carrie's Tip #3: Don't smoke. Quitting smoking is beyond the scope of this book, but I strongly urge you to do whatever it takes to break the habit.

If you do smoke, healthy eating is critical. Since smoking depletes Vitamin C from your body, you need to add more food containing this and other vital nutrients to your diet.

Oranges and orange juice.

Carrots and carrot juice.

Broccoli. Go ahead and drown it in processed cheese sauce if you have to make it more palatable.

Spinach. I'm not a huge fan of the taste, but eat it on subs along with every other vegetable the restaurant has to offer.

Kiwi.

Water. Drink enough water to hydrate yourself but don't go overboard as a friend's elderly mother did when her doctor told her to drink "lots of water." Too much of a good thing is a bad thing. Eight to ten glasses a day is tops.

Aunt Carrie's Tip #4. Be vigilant in caring for your teeth and gums. Poor hygiene can cause major problems in your general health, not to mention cause pain – and worse than that, it can make you look older than you are.

If you don't already have regular check-ups find a compatible dentist. I don't have dental insurance, so I frequent a university dental clinic where the students are closely supervised and the cost is about 50% of work done by a dentist in private practice. The visit takes longer because every step is monitored by a dental professor, but it's worth it to me.

Ask your dentist or hygienist to instruct you on proper home care. Yes, you've been brushing your teeth since you were two, but there might be a new technique or two that you need to learn.

Electric toothbrushes can be purchased from around $20 to over $100. I love the way mine ($20) massages my gums. Water pics are an alternative to twice daily flossing. I also recently found a tiny toothbrush, about the size of a dental pick, that cleans between teeth.

Aunt Carrie's Tip #5. Get a good night's sleep.

No caffeine after noon.

Don't drink too much water (or any other liquid) late in the day or you might have to get up and make a trip or two to the bathroom.

Although a moderate amount of alcohol is often recommended as a sleep aid, it wears off quickly and there you lay, wide awake. If you drink too much – well, you know. Hang-overs are not healthy.

Stop checking email an hour or two before bedtime.

Your bedroom is your own little piece of paradise so keep it clutter free (yes, we are all too tired at times to do anything other than drop our clothes on the floor and crawl into bed). Treat yourself to some pretty sheets.

Allowing your pet(s) into your bedroom can disrupt your sleep. Can? Does! Do I care? No. My dog and I have been through an empty nest, our pack leader dying leaving me a widow, thunderstorms, power outages, and a burglary.   I think that makes my beloved dog welcome to snooze anywhere he wants, and he happens to prefer my side of the bed.

Your bed is for sleeping and making love, not working, not worrying.

Keep a pen and paper next to your bed so that you can write down anything important that pops into your mind and not worry about remembering it the next morning. I send texts to myself: buy orange juice, call vet to make appointment, take cans to recycle bin.

Conventional wisdom demands you get out of bed and go to another room if you suffer from insomnia. I am lucky in that most nights I fall quickly to dreamland, but when I do have difficulty getting to sleep I either tell myself in a stern manner, "It is time to go to sleep" or I inhale deeply, hold my breath for a few seconds, then exhale. Rubbing the bottoms of my feet with mentholated petroleum jelly also seems to work.

Create a routine by going to bed and getting up the same time every day whenever possible.

Keep your bedroom comfy, quiet and dark. Since I do have pets I wash my sheets frequently. I also hang them (the bedding, not my dog and cats) outdoors to dry whenever possible.

If you absolutely must take a nap, remember that it could disturb your sleep patterns and you might end up with a touch of insomnia later that night.

Get as much natural light as you can. Go for a walk in the sunshine whenever possible.

Turn off your tv, computer and other electronic devices an hour or two before bedtime. The light they generate will keep you from falling asleep.

Use low wattage lights bulbs in your bedside lamps.

Get into a peaceful, relaxing bedtime routine. Take a bubble bath, have a small bowl of ice cream, drink hot cocoa, flip through a home and garden magazine filled with beautiful pictures, meditate on all the blessings bestowed upon you during the day. Pray, if you are a believer. Put all worries out of your mind. This is easier said than done, and I have lain awake worrying about finances more often than I care to remember. However, emulate a dog's behavior: if you can't eat it or play with it, urinate on it and go on your merry way. You can figure out money and other worries in the bright light of day when they aren't as scary.

Your bedroom should be quiet, but if it isn't, consider

drowning out noise (traffic, neighbors, dogs) with a white noise machine. If you don't have one, can't afford one, or don't know where to get a white noise machine, just turn on a fan.

A cool, not cold, bedroom promotes deep sleep. Keep an extra blanket at the foot of the bed in case you do get cold, and keep a fan handy if the warm is too hot and stuffy.

You need a comfortable bed. If yours is lumpy, consider investing in a good quality mattress and box springs. If you cannot afford a new bed, please think twice about bringing a used one into your home. If you think you can't afford a new bed, wait until you have to pay an exterminator to rid the place of bed buds. I've known two people whose homes were invaded by bedbugs. Both had clean houses. Both spent considerable time and money getting rid of the critters. Did you know that they not only get into bedding, clothing and other soft items but also into any available crevices, including under pictures, light switches and power outlets?

If you can't replace your bed at this time, invest in an egg crate topper.

Your bed should give you enough room to stretch out comfortable.

Hunger can keep you awake, but so can eating heavy meals late in the day. Here are a few sleep friendly snacks to tide you over under morning:

An apple

Banana

Turkey sandwich (save the spicy mustard for daytime)

A small bowl of cereal

Yogurt

Ice cream (my favorite)

Hot cocoa

Create a simple routine: wash face, brush teeth and apply hand lotion. For extra soft skin, wear lightweight moisturizing gloves overnight.

Spritz light cologne on your wrists for pleasant dreams.

An easy way to get to sleep – fast. Breathe in for four seconds; hold for seven seconds; then breathe out for eight seconds. This method was developed by a Harvard-educated, wellness practitioner. Dr. Andrew Weil specializes in breathing, meditation, and how it can be used to counteract stress. "…slows down your heart rate and it also releases chemicals in your brain that soothe you." I have used it and been shocked at how quickly I fell asleep. However, you should consult with your doctor before trying this since it slows down your heart.

Aunt Carrie's Tip No. 6: Forgive those who trespassed against you.

A man that studieth revenge keeps his own wounds green, which otherwise would heal and do well. Francis Bacon.

It's difficult, but if you hold on to resentment you are poisoning your soul and making yourself sick. You are not hurting the one who hurt you. In fact, there are some people who would be thrilled to think that they are important enough to continue controlling your emotions by their dirty deed(s).

In severe cases, you might have to get professional help in order to rid yourself of the burden of holding a grudge. In the case of egregious, aggressive and unwarranted behavior toward me, I know I would, because I am not Jesus and I don't have Alzheimer's.

Oh, even if you are successful in the ol' forgive, forget arena, be on guard against further attacks from the person. It's not "fool me once, shame on you; fool me twice, shame on me" because it is never your fault when someone humiliates you or steals from you or ruins your reputation or is physically aggressive. But even after a smiling truce, keep your distance.

Regardless of the situation, don't let hate eat you alive. Let go of the past and consider whatever went on between you to be the problem of the bully, gossip, liar or abuser and no longer your problem.

Aunt Carrie's Tip No. 7: And while you're at it, forgive yourself, too. Although it takes cojones, do what you can to make amends, if at all possible. Unfortunately, it often isn't. Perhaps the person is no longer living or you don't know how to contact her/him. Occasionally it is more sensible or kind to let sleeping dogs lie instead of stirring up the past. Apologizing to someone you stalked or asking forgiveness from the wife of a man with whom you had an affair could be construed as hostility concealed as concern.

If you do have the ability to ask forgiveness of someone you have wronged, be brave. Many will be pleasantly surprised to hear a heartfelt apology but a few might not be ready, willing or able to let the past rest, particularly if your trespass was egregious.

If you can't make it up to those you have wronged, pay it forward by donating time or money to a worthy cause. Since many charitable organizations have heavy overhead, you might want to do something more personal than writing a check so as to get as much bang for the buck as possible. I personally don't like my contributions going to administrative costs.

How about buying coats at Christmas time and donating them to a homeless shelter or to a coat drive? You don't have to spend a fortune, either. Several friends and I buy gently used coats. We also buy new toys and clothing at clearance sales throughout the year to be distributed through the Salvation Army. Food banks need their shelves restocked. (Skip the dented can bin.) Macaroni and cheese, canned tuna, peanut butter, cereal, condiments and boxed or canned milk are always appreciated.

Do it anonymously or give it in the first name of the person you've hurt or deceased relative or friend. You don't want to take credit for the generosity because you are paying a debt to make up for past indiscretions.

Aunt Carrie's Tip No. 8: Give of yourself. Grandma Helen was shy and not much of a joiner, but she enjoyed her volunteer job at the Red Cross Blood Drive. She got dressed up, manned the intake desk and socialized with women she would not have otherwise known.

Yours truly started volunteering when she was stuck in a dead-end job, complete with two bullies, in hopes that being around other like minded people would save her sanity.

I read inspirational works to the visually impaired for five years, reluctantly quitting when there were too many demands on my time when I was widowed and had to take a second job.

For most of my adult life I have volunteered for animal rescue groups, learning to build websites and marketing our fund-raisers. In return, I get help with veterinarian bills and pet food, and fellow volunteers have become family.

Two years ago I was able to carve out a few hours a week to volunteer at a sheltered workshop. Although in theory I am "helping" others, I am the one who benefits from working with these so-called "disabled" adults. Although they are learning job skills, they also are teaching me patience, kindness and gratitude.

A compassionate and fun loving friend excitedly told me about her new volunteer job with Make a Wish Foundation. She and a partner (no one is ever alone with a child to avoid any accusations of improprieties or danger to the volunteer) make a home visit and fill out a questionnaire so that they can recommend a child be granted his or her wish. A six year old and his family are going to fly to Disney World and ride in a limo to and from the park, something they could never afford on their own. Amy said that she was afraid she might be sad, but instead she enjoys working with families of critically ill children.

There are many other worthy causes that need what you have to offer. If interested, visit http://www.volunteermatch.org to find a cause close to your heart.

Aunt Carrie's Tip #9. Be grateful. Meditate or pray. Every night before you go to sleep, count your blessings. If this strikes you as too spiritual, then write a list, practically speaking. "Today I had enough money to buy groceries…put gasoline in the car…I have a comfortable bed…a roof over my head…electricity…" No matter what your circumstances, many people would trade places with you in a heartbeat.

Be grateful for your health. Most of us can walk, talk, see, hear.

Give thanks for family and friends.

Honor Mother Nature's bounty by recycling if possible. If you can't, you can perhaps appreciate flowers and trees and all of creation.

As we speak, a ten year old lilac is blooming outside my window. Last year Jack Frost nipped it before it could blossom, so today I am thankful for the florets which seem exceptionally colorful and the delightful scent. Even the delivery man commented on the fragrance as he walked up to the house.

Aunt Carrie's Tip #10: Enjoy little luxuries. Why live a long life if you don't have a little fun along the way?

Indulge yourself with a little luxury of your choice. It should be something like makes you feel spoiled, but still needs to be within your budget.

Fine china is frequently available at thrift stores and yard sales. You can mix and match pieces as your collection grows. Heat water in a china tea pot, then steep imported tea in a matching cup. Savor.

Spoil yourself with bouquets of fresh cut flowers. If you have a green thumb, consider growing an unusual plant, or at the very least something that not everyone has. Orchids are fussy, but worth the maintenance.

Buy a bottle of ridiculously expensive wine and have a shot on special occasions.

I like changing my sheets every other day, especially during warm weather when they are able to line dry and soak up the sun.

You might like to use a fancy pen.

A warm bath is a luxurious way to end the day. Sometimes I pour in a little Epsom salt along with bubble bath.

You don't have to be told that a few pieces of your favorite candy can be quite luxurious.

Aunt Carrie's Tip #11: Get involved with a hobby.

Hobbies and interests can make you happy. Even if your only interest is watching tv, find a show that you truly enjoy.   Two of my guilty pleasures are Law and Order: Special Victims Unit and Mayberry re-runs (decades old, in black and white, with the unforgettable Barney Fife).

Do you like bargain shopping? House plants? Going to classic car shows? Thrift stores? Sports?

One acquaintance collects bricks. At first, this seemed a little odd (boring), but after going to a demonstration of 1800 brick making (from straw and mud) and then reading about brick factories of the early 1900s and their names imprinted in them, I developed an interest. I now have two, both of historic nature, and will be looking for more.

Aunt Carrie's Tip 12: Look young, feel young.

Thinking young is one of the best ways to stay young and healthy for as long as possible. Thinking young doesn't mean making a spectacle of yourself by wearing clothing appropriate for a teen-ager. However, dressing a decade or two younger is much more flattering than looking like someone's grandmother even if you are a Grandma Helen or even Great-Grandma Helen.

A middle-aged friend still is into mother-daughter

lookalike clothing. She and Mom shop together and buy pantsuits from an upscale department store. Mom doesn't look a day younger and unfortunately Daughter looks twenty years older than her chronological age.

Wear flattering colors. Aqua is universally refreshing, youthful and feminine. We don't mean to be sexist, so if you are a guy know that almost any shade of blue will compliment your good looks.

Bright colors lighten the mood and pastels look good on some, but wash out others. Determine which shade of pink favors your complexion, and wear it often. Watermelon is a good choice for most of us. Hot pink is "mine" but salmon makes me look ill.

If your wardrobe consists of mostly black or other neutrals, add colorful scarves and accessories and eventually replace most of the duller clothing with red, green, orange, blue and purple apparel. You will want and need a few black items and perhaps a few shades of brown.

Nothing is more aging that wearing too much jewelry, especially matched sets. Tiny earrings are more youthful than large. While rings can add to your look, don't wear more too many or anything too large. Your hands and nails should be neatly manicured and creamed. A light pink or clear nail polish is more youthful than bright red. If your hands are chapped or old looking, please don't draw attention to them.

Light, fruity colognes are young and flirty so leave heavier perfumes to women who want to appear matronly.

Another important way to look and feel younger is to update your hairstyle. Tightly permed curls are particularly aging. Ask your stylist to make your hair loose and free.

When I told a friend I was getting a make-over at a local teaching salon, she worried that I would be wearing the current "over forty" look, but fortunately I don't follow the crowd. Although short hair is considered youthful, it doesn't work for me. The point is – wear your hair any length you like.

Layers allow your hair to swing, giving you a young look. Bangs hide wrinkles around your eyes and on your forehead.

Curling irons and blow driers do add style and volume, but they also damage hair, which is not a young look. Although you can protect your hair by applying product (conditioners, mouse), they build up and you can end up with lank, drooping locks. A simple cut will allow you to do away with setting lotions, hot rollers, flat irons, curling irons, curl boosting jellies and mousses. A style that allows a natural air dry is especially important if you color your hair. Too much teasing and chemicals can cause damage that can only be remedied by cutting inches off your precious locks.

Hair color is the easier way to erase years from your appearance. Although gray hair can be gorgeous on some women, it more often shouts a woman is no longer young and has lost interest in her looks. Adding highlights or lowlights gives hair depth and shine. If your hair is naturally dark brown or black, it is especially important to weave in highlights so as to avoid the Shoe Polish Look. Unrelieved dark hair is a harsh, hard look.

Keep color alive and vibrant by using shampoo and conditioner formulated for tinted hair.

Wear make-up lightly applied but with a hint of color. Sparkle with a pink glossy lipstick and liquid blush blended into your cheeks.

Moisturizer is one of our best friends. Apply to your

face and neck, into your chest, after your morning shower and again at night after removing your make-up.

Moisturizing hand cream is a must for youthful looking hands. Wearing cotton moisturizing gloves over smoothly creamed hands is an inexpensive and easy overnight beauty treatment. You can also wear them under garden gloves during the day.

You don't have to be reminded to use rubber or plastic gloves any time you immerse your hands in a harsh cleaning solution.

There are several methods of removing facial hair so you might want to experiment until you find one that works best for you. Hot wax seems to be more effective than cold. Mustaches and whiskers sprouting out of a woman's chin is not the look you are after. Some women bleach facial hair but a lightened mustache is still a mustache.

Foundation make-up will not cover up facial hair but will instead draw attention to it.

Diamonds might be said to be a girl's best friend, but I prefer a pair of tweezers and carry them with me everywhere I go. If you see a dizzy blonde sitting at a traffic light, pluck, pluck, plucking away, wave and say hi. Tweezing is particularly effective on the hair sprouting on our chinny chin chins. When I'm feeling adventurous I yank out hair above my lips.

Epilators work well, pulling out multiple hairs at once, but the procedure is too painful for me. Epilators are not costly so you might want to give one a try.

Chemical depilatories dissolve unwanted hair. They are easy to use, inexpensive to buy and pain free. Follow directions closely to avoid chemical burns.

In times of desperation I have shaved my mustache.

It's not ideal, but it is fast and effective. Toss out dull razor blades. They pull, not trim, leaving marks on your face.

Laser hair removal uses light to destroy hair roots. Laser removal is most effective with light skin and dark hair, which leaves me out because although my skin is light, so is my facial hair (gray).

Electrolysis destroys hair growth by inserting a tiny needle into the skin. Consult a dermatologist to see if laser hair removal or electrolysis is suitable for your skin and hair type.

Keep up with the latest trends. Learn new skills. Consider enrolling in an adult education class. Listen to new music. That seems to be hard for many of us as we seem to be stuck in a decade when all the music was good as opposed to the junk being recorded today. Reality check! The songs of our youth were not all good and there are a few current ones worth listening to. Follow a new group or singer.

Styles in books change over the years. Find a new author and maybe even a new to you genre.

I personally am guilty of this. Don't tell and retell the same stories over and over, especially ones that make you sound judgmental. Judgmental is old. You are committed to staying young.

If you feel silly using current slang, don't force it. However, drop the old. "Sharp" was cool in 1966. It's no longer 1966.

Exercise will keep you younger.   You will have better posture and you will have more energy.

Incorporating fruits and vegetables into your diet will brighten your complexion.

Romance (or sex) is another way to Think Young. If

you have a partner, enjoy your relationship, and if you don't, take a chance and look for love.

Smile! Happy equals younger. Regular dental care will keep you lookin' good – and younger.

If you have a question about your make-up, hair color, clothing style or jewelry, ask yourself if Mrs. Roper of Three's Company fame would wear it. If she would, you have your answer. It is not for you.

Aunt Carrie's Tip 13: Playing it safe -- on the information superhighway.

Do not give personal contact information or anything that could reveal hints about where you live, your occupation when filling out your profile on dating websites. Give a little thought to your email address. Greeneyes@whatever.com is cute and clean; 2sexyxxx is not.

If a man mentions "destiny," "fate" or "soul mate" early on, he might be a hit and run guy. He also might be interested in taking you for a wild ride, financially.

If he is "recently widowed" he could be trouble. Either he is lying in an attempt to gain your sympathy and confidence or he is telling the truth and that could be just as bad. It is common for widowers to still be married (in their hearts) to their deceased wife. "She was an angel," "I treated her like the angel she was," and "Our marriage was perfect" are all things widowers have said to me. Even though I myself am widowed, I prefer divorced men, as they seem more rational. Do you really want to be compared with an angel?

Whether it is a date or meeting to conduct a sale of merchandise, meet in a well lighted, public place. The mall, a casual restaurant or coffee shop is the perfect venue for a first date. Take time to know your potential romantic partner before going to his house or even telling him where you live.

I did not give a date my home address and did not like it when he told me that he had google mapped my house (using my phone number). His excuse? Women who lived in "crappy" apartments that were after his money. That was our first and last date. There may be gold diggers out there, but I am not one. I am considering getting a cheap cell phone that can be used just for dating purposes until I find the right guy.

Let a friend or relative know the name of the man you are meeting, the place, and approximately how long you will be out. Provide your own transportation, to and from your date. First dates shouldn't last hours and hours, no matter how smitten you are. Also, have someone call you while you are out, so that he will know that at least one person is aware of your whereabouts. You might want to have a safe word, something to let your friend know that no, you are not ok. It shouldn't be anything unusual so as to tip off your date. How about mentioning your dog, real or imaginary, to alert your friend, "I need help getting out of this situation."

You don't need to be reminded that you should not drink. One: alcohol can cloud your otherwise good judgment and you might end up in bed on your first date (horrible idea). Two: you need to remain sober because you are driving home.

If you are involved in a long distance romance, your first date is going to be even trickier, because you are not going to be alone with him during your initial visit. Remember – you do not know this man. You are not staying at his house. This means you will check into a hotel (not a motel, but an upscale hotel with security). If you flew to meet your date, you will need to rent your own car. If this is too expensive, perhaps you should re-think your relationship. It goes without saying that if he comes to your location, he will have to provide his own lodging.   Have someone know your schedule.

Observe the above precautions that you would take when meeting a local man: provide your own transportation to and from your dates, have someone call you, don't drink. Yes, this sounds boring, and yes, love is an adventure, but you still need to stay safe.

When meeting someone new, always, always, always trust your instincts. If he seems too good to be true, he probably is. If you think he is lying (about anything), beware.

Protect your finances. If you receive an email requesting money, delete the message. No, your daughter is not being held in jail in a foreign country and the only way she can be released is if you wire her money.

Aunt Carrie's Tip 14: Play it safe in real life: common sense outdoor safety tips.   In order to live a long and healthy life, you need to take care to prevent accidents.

Although Grandma Helen never mowed the grass, I have, many times, so I am qualified to give you a little lawn worthy advice.

Wear sturdy shoes while using a lawn mower

Turn off mower and let blades stop spinning before removing grass from blades

Keep children inside while you are mowing

Grilling – even girls can do it

Grills are for outdoor use only.

Keep grills at least ten feet from your house, tree branches and deck railing.

Don't allow children or pets to play near the grill.

Never pour gasoline on the grill.

Have a garden hose nearby.

Grandma Helen was not a sun worshipper. These tips are from her.

If you sunburn easily, stay indoors between 10 a.m. and 4 p.m.

Drink plenty of water to prevent heat exhaustion and dehydration

Wear sun block, a wide brimmed hat and sunglasses. I wish you can have seen my mother, wearing large sunglasses and a big straw hat with multicolored band with multicolored ribbon flapping in the wind as she flew down the road in her Ford Torino. She also wore SPF 15 sunscreen anytime she left the house, and I do mean anytime, if only to retrieve something from the car.

Protect yourself during thunder storms.

Seek indoor shelter during lightning storms, leaving golf clubs, aluminum baseball bats and fishing poles behind.

Do not use electric appliances or phones. Grandma Helen often told me to hang up the landline, believing lightning would flow through the wire and electrocute me. She was right – who knew?

If you have a jacket, take it off and put it under your feet to insulate you.

My good friend Karina's mother was much like mine. Whenever she saw a newspaper article about a weather related death, she would circle it with a red pen and mail it to her daughter. Karina kept the picture of cows struck down in a Midwestern field.

Traffic safety is probably the most important because it is likely driving is an everyday occurrence. Whether you like it or not, you need to buckle up whenever you are in a car, no matter how short the trip.

Distracted driving kills. Don't text, don't talk on your cell phone, don't change CDs, don't eat, don't smoke, don't check your make-up. Don't, don't, don't. I've seen people reading while driving 60 mph and women applying lipstick.

Drive defensively.

Do you see the signs on the highway with a phone number to report an impaired driver? This means all of us – don't drink and drive, don't drive while under the influence of any drug, street or pharmaceutical, don't drive while emotionally upset. If you are impaired, call a friend, call a cab, or sleep it off in your car.

Stay alert. Don't drive when sleepy or too tired to handle the responsibility of operating a motor vehicle. Stop and stretch your legs or have a soft drink if you are on a trip.

Keep your car well maintained. Good tires and brakes in working condition are only two of the things you need for a safe drive. If your car overheats or stalls, you could get stuck in traffic – and struck by traffic.

Obey the law. If you frequently get stopped for speeding, learn to shut it down. Comply with all other rules of the road. If it's been awhile since you took driver's training, pick up a driving booklet geared for those getting their licenses for the first time at the DMV and refresh your memory.

Honk your horn only when absolutely necessary. Remember that there are people carrying loads guns in their vehicles and some of them are unstable and looking for a slight and an excuse for a fight.

Avoid eye contact with drivers who might be angry with you. Yes, you might be in the right, but do you want to be dead right?

Never flip the bird to another driver. You didn't have to be told that, did you? I had to learn the hard way to keep my emotions in check. When my kids were toddlers, years before road rage was A Thing, a young guy cut me off. Instead of being responsible and ignoring the incident, I gave him the finger. He pulled in front of me, stopped his car, tried to block me and got out, slamming his door and storming toward our car. I was able to get around him and I took off.

Don't tailgate.

Give reckless drivers plenty of room. I stay well behind cars that are swerving and don't attempt to pass them no matter how slow they are driving.

Adjust your mirrors so that they give you the best view.

Keep headlights clean.

Car kit:

Spare tire (I've never learned to change one but I have one for the roadside assistance crew)

Roadside assistance. I get mine with my cell phone package. $4 a month provides security in knowing that someone will help me when I need it.

Jumper cables.

First aid kit.

A fully charged cell phone.

Flashlight with working batteries.

Bottled water.

Blanket.

Warm jacket or coat.

Fix a Flat.

A quart or two of motor oil.

Gallon of antifreeze.

Ice scraper.

Paper and pen.

Life as a pedestrian.

Carry a fully charged cell phone, but be aware of your surroundings instead of wandering the streets with your phone at your ear.

In kindergarten we learned, "Stop, look and listen before you cross the street. Use your eyes, use your ears, before you use your feet." When crossing a street, never assume that every driver will stop for a red light. A mailman once pushed me out of the way of a distracted driver, saying that he dodges traffic regularly and a red light means nothing to some.

Aunt Carrie's Tip #15: Play it safe - but not too safe.

Clean is great, but a little dirt never hurt anyone – and

can help build your immune system. So if you like the Great Outdoors, indulge yourself. Dig into the dirt and plant a flower.

If someone asks you out, and you want to go, go. Be careful, of course, but not too careful. Life is a risk and so is love.

If you hate your job (and haven't we all at one time?), look for another. Even in these rough financial times, take a step out of your cocoon (with a nest egg) and see where you land. Don't quit your day job until you have solid employment, though. In the meantime, turn a hobby into a career or work as a volunteer until you can finagle a paying gig. Also, don't take on debt, personal or business, during your transition period. To impress a prospective employer, take a course or two outside the job description. If you can do a little programming, or web design, or creative or technical writing, you will be miles ahead of competitors.

If you have always wanted to learn to swim, learn to speak another language, learn to dance, learn to paint, become an auxiliary police officer, start your own business, get married, get divorced, change religion, decorate your home, build a better wardrobe, dye your hair – whatever – do it! In some instances (starting your own business) it would be best to start small and build as you go along, but jump in if you want to learn to swim.

Life is all around. Partake.

Conclusion:

If you take nothing else from this, remember:

Drink plenty of water.

Walk whenever possible.

Limit red meat.

Whenever possible choose foods with few additives.

Eat your vegetables!

If you don't like vegetables, find ways to sneak them into your diet.

Fruit is a very tasty way to nourish your body.

Nourish your soul by practicing the art of gratitude.

Never buy, or use, any food that comes in a can that is dented. Recently a local woman died of botulism.

Keep your cool.

Avoid unnecessary stress.

Avoid debt. Everyone might want a fancy house or car but not everyone's budget might not allow the finer things in life – at this time. There is always the future. Fortunes do change.

Illegitimi non carborundum.   (Don't let the bastards drag you down).